GASTROPARESIS DIET

Delicious, Nutritious Recipes for Gastro paresis Relief

Joseph J. Lucas

Table of Contents

CHAPTER 1
WHAT IS GASTROPARESIS

Gastro paresis is an problem in which your tummy gets rid of into your little intestinal tract machine extra gradually in comparison to it must.

Gastro paresis may be precipitated with the aid of using a situation or an enduring fitness trouble, consisting of diabetic problems mellitus or lupus.

Symptoms and symptoms and symptoms are probably mild or

enormous and normally comprise:

- tossing up
- bloating
- nausea or vomiting or throwing up
- heartburn

Commonly gastro paresis is a temporary indicator that the frame has honestly every other factor which you`re managing. Oftentimes it is a relentless, or lasting, trouble.

Gastro paresis can further arise after bariatric clinical remedy or every other expert remedy that interrupts your meals digestion.

When you've got honestly gastro paresis, the quantity of fat and fiber which you absorb can dramatically have an impact on simply how extreme your signs and symptoms and symptoms are. Dietary modifications are normally the at the beginning method of remedy cautioned to human beings which have honestly actually gastro paresis.

If you've got honestly simply gastro paresis, it is crucial to attention on obtaining the vitamins which you name for even as taking in little, non-stop food which might be decreased in fats and primary to absorb.

Among one of the maximum crucial ingredients on this sort of weight loss plan routine ordinary comprise excessive healthful and balanced healthful protein ingredients (consisting of eggs and velvety nut butter) and easy-to-digest greens (consisting of prepared zucchini).

If the meals is primary to devour and devour, it really is an first rate indicator that you'll have honestly an simpler time taking in it.

Here's a imparting of cautioned ingredients that would assist maintain your gastro paresis in check:

- eggs
- clean or velvety peanut butter
- bananas
- white breads, decreased fiber or fine-tuned cereals, and narrow biscuits
- fruit juice
- veggie juice (spinach, kale, carrots)
- fruit purees

If you presently have honestly gastro paresis signs and symptoms and symptoms, it is crucial to renowned what ingredients to stay loose from.

As an essential plan, ingredients which might be excessive in fats or fiber must absolutely be taken in little amounts.

Here's a imparting of ingredients that would make your gastro paresis pain additionally even worse:

- carbonated beverages
- alcohol

- beans and legumes

- corn

- seeds and nuts

- broccoli and cauliflower

- cheese

- massive cream

- unwanted oil or butter

When you are improving from a gastro paresis flare-up, you may have honestly to gain on a multiphase weight loss plan routine ordinary that regularly reintroduces stable ingredients.

While there aren't any government weight loss plan

routine ordinary necessities for gastro paresis flares, a variety of human beings locate it crucial to conform with a three-section weight loss plan routine ordinary.

The three levels are as adheres to:
- Originally section. You're restrained in particular to combination or bouillon soups, further to incorporated veggie juice.
- 2d section. You may paintings round soups which encompass biscuits and noodles, further to cheese and velvety peanut butter.

- 0.33 sections. You're made it viable for to have honestly maximum of soft, easy-to-chunk starches, further to softer healthful and balanced healthful protein reasserts consisting of chook and fish.

Throughout all levels of this healing weight loss plan routine ordinary, it is crucial to stay loose from pork and excessive fiber greens considering that they take loads longer to absorb.

When you've got honestly gastro paresis, you must attempt to recollect simply how normally and in what buy you devour ingredients. It's endorsed you're taking in little food, five to eight instances every day.

Consume your meals nicely within side the preceding eating it. Take in useful ingredients at the beginning to stay loose from bearing on be complete from ingredients that do not fuelling your frame.

While improving from gastro paresis, reflect on consideration on taking a multivitamin complement so that you can nevertheless get the vitamins you name for. If weight lower changed into an illustration of your gastro paresis, go together with a marginal of 1,500 energy everyday as you starting your healing.

Nutritional beverages are easy-to-digest beverages that may assist with this. These comprise:

- yogurt smoothies
- fruit and veggie smoothies
- liquid meal opportunity beverages

- healthful and balanced healthful protein beverages

Take in notable offers of spray so your meals digestion machine would not get dehydrated.

Remain loose from alcohol if you have honestly gastro paresis signs and symptoms and symptoms, as alcohol can dehydrate or constipate you added — together with decrease your ranges of precise vitamins.

Meals

Your meals alternatives may honestly simply sense restrained if you have honestly gastro paresis, though you may nevertheless price a few scrumptious food.

Peach banana smoothies and inexperienced smoothies with peanut butter comprise the vitamins you name for and desire outstanding.

For mouthwatering alternatives, garlic mashed potatoes and gastro paresis-pleasant veggie soup have honestly little bit fiber though top offers of desire.

Takeaway

While gastro paresis is normally relentless, it could be short-lived occasionally. It may be an illustration of every other trouble, or it could be idiopathic, which recommends the expand is unidentified.

Despite what the expand or length of your gastro paresis, taking in little food and proscribing your fiber and fats utilization can assist your meals digestion.

Numerous human beings with several diagnoses can maintain precise meals factors higher in comparison to others. Continuously speak with a medical doctor or dietitian pertaining on your individualized dietary wishes even as dealing with gastro paresis.

It's crucial to assure your frame continues to be obtaining the minerals and nutrients wanted for healthful and balanced and stabilized frame organ run as you redeem out of your gastro paresis signs and symptoms and symptoms.

CHAPTER 2

DIABETIC MAN OR WOMAN CHARACTER GASTROPARESIS

Gastro paresis, further referred to as held off gastric emptying, is a trouble of the meals digestion machine that produces meals to constantly continue to be within side the tummy for a quantity of time it really is loads longer in comparison to normal.

This happens because the nerves that switch meals with the meals digestion machine are damaged, so muscle tissues mass do not paintings properly.

Subsequently, meals beings within side the tummy undigested.

Among one of the maximum common foundation aid of gastro paresis is diabetic problems mellitus. It can expand and development with time, especially in people with out of control blood glucose diploma ranges.

In this write-up, we will cowl the concepts of gastro paresis, containing signs and symptoms and symptoms, evasion, and extra.

The abiding with the aid of using are signs and symptoms and symptoms of gastro paresis:

- heartburn
- nausea or vomiting or throwing up
- tossing up of undigested meals
- extraordinarily very early amount after a piece meal
- weight lower
- bloating
- anorexia nervosa
- blood glucose ranges which might be tough to maintain

- tummy spasms
- acid reflux

Gastro paresis signs and symptoms and symptoms is probably little or enormous, counting on the Parkinson`s disorder constant pancreatitis cystic fibrosis kidney disorde

Turner condition

Typically no stated expand can probably lie, after substantial testing.

Origin assets of gastro paresis

People which have actually gastro paresis have issues to their vague nerve. This prevents nerve run in addition to meals digestion for the reason that impulses had to churn meals are reduced or stop. Gastro paresis is tough to identify in addition to consequently usually be going undiagnosed.

Gastro paresis is greater everyday in humans which have actually excessive, out of control blood sugar stage tiers over a extended quantity of time. Long time period intervals of excessive sugar within side the blood expand nerve issues all through the frame.

Persistently excessive blood sugar stage diploma tiers

moreover issues the capillary that supply the frame's nerves in addition to frame organs with sustenance in addition to oxygen. This carries the vague nerve in addition to meals digestion machine, each which in some unspecified time in the future reason gastro paresis.

Since gastro paresis is a colorful disorder, in addition to multiple of its signs and symptoms and symptoms and symptoms like constant heartburn or queasiness or throwing up display up every day, you won't understand which you have the hassle.

When meals isn't always honestly really digested typically, it may probably constantly continue to be within side the tummy, triggering signs and symptoms and symptoms and symptoms of amount in addition to bloating. Undigested meals can probably moreover create stable hundreds referred to as bezoars that may probably make contributions to:

- queasiness or throwing up
- tossing up
- clog of the little intestines

Gastro paresis materials substantial issues for humans with diabetic troubles mellitus considering the fact those hold-ups in meals digestion make coping with blood sugar stage challenging.

The disorder makes the meals digestion remedy hard to track, so sugar analyses can probably remodel. If you've got got really honestly choppy sugar analyses, percentage them together along with your health practitioner, in conjunction with diverse different signs and symptoms and symptoms and symptoms you are experiencing.

Gastro paresis is a constant issue, in addition to having really honestly the hassle can probably really honestly sense aggravating.

Undertaking the remedy of producing nutritional adjustments in addition to proceeding to govern blood sugar stage diploma tiers at the same time as feeling ill in addition to nauseated to the variable of tossing up is laborious. Those with gastro paresis usually really honestly sense worsened in addition to medically clinically depressed.

Your health practitioner will honestly in reality do not forget quite a few factors within side the preceding locating you with diabetic character person gastro paresis. They'll do not forget your expert records in addition to signs and symptoms and symptoms and symptoms, in addition to execute a bodily examination to attempt to locate signs of gastro paresis. Indicators can also additionally encompass:

- belly
- location
- swelling or pain

- dehydration

- insufficient nourishment

Your health practitioner may moreover gather blood or pee reviews to attempt to locate any sort of form of troubles of gastro paresis. Imaging reviews may moreover be made use to attempt to locate any sort of form of tummy blockages.

A couple of diverse different reviews your health practitioner may execute encompass esophagogastroduodenoscopy or gastric emptying scintigraphy.

An

esophagogastroduodenoscopy

can probably plan out infections in addition to decide the presence of any sort of form of meals left within side the tummy. Gastric emptying scintigraphy is a machine made use for studying gastric emptying. It's taken into consideration the gold conventional within side the scientific analysis of gastro paresis.

Treatment of gastro paresis

Your health practitioner will honestly in reality moreover greater than possibly remodel your insulin application as needed. They may advise the following:

- taking insulin greater frequently or converting the sort of insulin you take
- taking insulin after recipes, in evaluation to withinside the preceding
- studying blood sugar stage tiers automatically after taking in in addition to taking insulin whilst needed

Your health practitioner will honestly in reality have the ability to present you greater unique requirements on how whilst to take your insulin.

Gastro paresis, additionally referred to as not on time gastric emptying, is a hassle of the belly machine that units off meals to constantly continue to be within side the belly for a quantity of time this is loads longer in comparison with regular.

This takes place for the reason that nerves that removal meals with the belly machine are damaged, so muscle groups mass do not paintings properly. Subsequently, meals beings within side the belly undigested.

Among one of the maximum everyday beginning aid of gastro paresis is diabetic troubles mellitus. It can absolutely expand in conjunction with development slowly, mainly in people with unrestrained blood sugar stage diploma tiers.

In this quick post, we're going to cowl the fundamentals of gastro paresis, containing signs and symptoms and symptoms and symptoms, evasion, in conjunction with greater.

symptoms of gastro paresis

- heartburn

- queasiness or throwing up

- tossing up of undigested meals

- honestly very early amount after a small meal

- weight monitoring

- bloating

- anorexia nervosa

- blood sugar stage tiers which are hard to keep

- belly spasms

acid reflux disease disorder

Gastro paresis signs and symptoms and symptoms might be little or severe, depending upon the issues to the vagus nerve, a extended cranial nerve that will increase from the brainstem to the stomach frame organs, containing the ones of the belly machine.

Symptoms and symptoms and symptoms can absolutely flare up any time, despite the fact that are greater every day after using excessive-fiber or excessive-fast foods, all which can be slow-shifting to soak up.

Girls with diabetic troubles mellitus have a excessive hazard for growing gastroparesis. Different diverse different troubles can absolutely fabric your hazard of growing the hassle, containing preceding tummy surgical procedures or records of taking in troubles.

Ailment in conjunction with troubles aside from diabetic troubles mellitus can absolutely expand gastroparesis, like:

- viral infections
- acid reflux disease disorder

- easy muscle cells troubles

- Parkinson's disorder
- constant pancreatitis
- cystic fibrosis
- kidney disorder
- Turner condition

Typically no stated expand can absolutely lie, after substantial testing.

Factors for gastroparesis

People which have gastroparesis have issues to their vagus nerve. This prevents nerve run in conjunction with meals meals digestion for the reason that impulses want to churn meals are decreased or stop. Gastro paresis is tough to decide in conjunction with therefore normally is going undiagnosed.

Gastro paresis is greater everyday in humans which have excessive, unrestrained blood sugar stage tiers over a extended amount of time. Comprehensive intervals of excessive sugar withinside the blood expand nerve issues all through the frame.

Frequently excessive blood sugar stage diploma tiers additionally issues the capillary that supply the frame's nerves in conjunction with frame organs with sustenance in conjunction with oxygen. This carries the vagus nerve in conjunction with belly machine, each which in some unspecified time in the future causes gastro paresis.

Since gastro paresis is a colorful disorder, in conjunction with multiple of its signs and symptoms and fats loss changes in blood sugar stage diploma levels

sizeable dehydration

esophagitis, or swelling of the
esophagus

absence of nourishment from
now no longer saturating up
nutrients

A lot of those signs and
symptoms and symptoms and
symptoms can truly intrude
together along with your manner
of living. A gastric emptying look
at can truly guide your physician
spot gastro paresis or special
diverse different motility hassle
triggering those signs and
symptoms and symptoms and
symptoms.

What to go away the remedy

Gastric emptying examines are completed at scientific facilities via way of means of professionals determined out nuclear drug or radiology.

Formerly the look at, you'll really absorb some thing solid (commonly clambered eggs), something liquid, and additionally a percentage of tasteless radioactive object. The radioactive product permits the virtual video cam to stick to the meals with the meals digestion treatment.

Then you'll really press a desk whilst the virtual video cam takes snap shots. Throughout three to five hrs, the virtual video cam will really take four to six examines long-lasting referring to a mins each. Some scientific facilities employ a gamma virtual video cam that takes snap shots whilst you`re standing. In both circumstance, it is critical to constantly be nonetheless during the look at.

Gastric emptying examines in younger humans

Gastro paresis signs and symptoms and symptoms and symptoms in younger humans appear to be the ones visible in grownups. Ask your physician to deliver this evaluation on your teen if they are experiencing any kind of amongst signs and symptoms and symptoms and symptoms cited previously.

The evaluation for older younger humans resembles the evaluation supplied to grownups. If your teen is a teen or infant, your physician offers your teen the radioactive meals in milk or system in an assessment referred to as a milk take a look at out or liquid take a look at out. In this situation, you will be endorsed to convey your man or woman system or milk from house to assure your teen does not have an allergic reaction.

The radioactive product is simply as as secure in your teen as it's miles for a grownup. The evaluation commonly takes pertaining to a few hrs for younger humans. If your teen is obtainable the liquid take a look at out instead, the virtual digital digital digicam takes non-stop snap shots for referring to a human resources. It's critical that the positive teen stays to be nonetheless during the evaluation. Guarantee which you situate a manner to continuously preserve them inhabited or relieve previously and during the evaluation to make sure that the give up consequences may be supplied successfully. The abiding via way of means of factors may want to guide maintain your teen unwinded:

- tracks
- playthings
- movie
- magazines
- ease factors, such coverings or pillows

You revel in a part of radiation immediately direct publicity from the object withinside the meals you devour previously your look at. This isn't always clearly really notion of dangerous except you are breast-feeding, expectant, or prep paintings to wound up being expectant. Anyone in those troubles must notify her physician previously having truly in truth a gastric emptying look at.

How you could put together

Besides the radioactive recipe previously the look at, you have to now no longer devour or devour something for four to six hrs previously the evaluation. If you've got got truely in truth diabetic man or woman issues, convey your medicines or insulin in situation your physician desires which you take them with the evaluation.

It's an outstanding thought to convey magazines or tracks to by skip the minute. A moms and daddy may want to preference to convey their kid's preferred plaything or pacifier.

Enable the professional pick out in case you are taking any kind of sort of medicines. The abiding via way of means of medicines can all impact exactly how quick your tummy receives rid of:

prokinetic sellers that boost up your meals digestion device

Antispasmodic sellers that decrease your meals digestion device

opioids, consisting of codeine, Norco, Percocet, and OxyContin

Health and wellbeing and fitness issues, consisting of diabetic man or woman issues or hypoglycemia, can impact the performance of the evaluation.

Your hormone representatives can moreover impact your evaluation give up consequences, so permit your physician in case you're within side the 2nd 1/2 of of your menstruation cycle.

Alternatives

Your physician may want to moreover use several diverse different checks to find out gastro paresis, containing:

a breath evaluation, wherein you devour a recipe organized with a particular sort of carbon and deliver breath times each quantity of hrs to make sure that the physician can look at its parts

the Smart Pill, an digital pill which you consume, which trips together along with your meals digestion device and sends information to a information receiver which you maintain with you during the evaluation

an ultrasound, that can permit your physician to peer your meals digestion device and select out whether or not some thing except gastro paresis is triggering your signs and symptoms and symptoms and symptoms a main belly (GI) endoscopy, wherein your physician uses an endoscope to peer your esophagus, tummy, and the start of your bit intestinal tract device to attempt to locate gastro paresis or blockage

a main GI collection, wherein you devour barium (which is simple to put on an X-ray) and feature a group of X-rays taken of your bit intestinal tract device

Talk on your physician pertaining to those options when you have truly in truth issues referring to the gastric emptying evaluation.

What to put together for after the evaluation

The physician that obtained the evaluation commonly telecellsmartphone calls inside some days with give up consequences.

Your physician may want to advocate medicines consisting of metoclopramide (Reglan), erythromycin, or antiemetics to control your gastro paresis and its signs and symptoms and symptoms and symptoms. They may want to moreover propose gastric electric enjoyment. In this remedy, a touch bit tool referred to as a gastric neurostimulator is surgically located into your stomach location to promote it the stomach muscular tissues mass. This is commonly endorsed really in case you do not reply to medicines.

In unusual, sizeable scenarios, you can want a jejunostomy. In this remedy, your physician inserts a feeding tube together along with your stomach location into the jejunum, part of your bit intestinal tract device. This remedy is really finished in case your gastro paresis is sizeable and has truly in truth a big effect in your manner of living.

For one of the maximum components, figuring out and managing gastro paresis previously any kind of sort of massive signs and symptoms and symptoms and symptoms show up creates a ideal outcome.

THE END